Thriving with chronic obstructive pulmonary disease COPD

Women's Journey to Wellness

Charles John

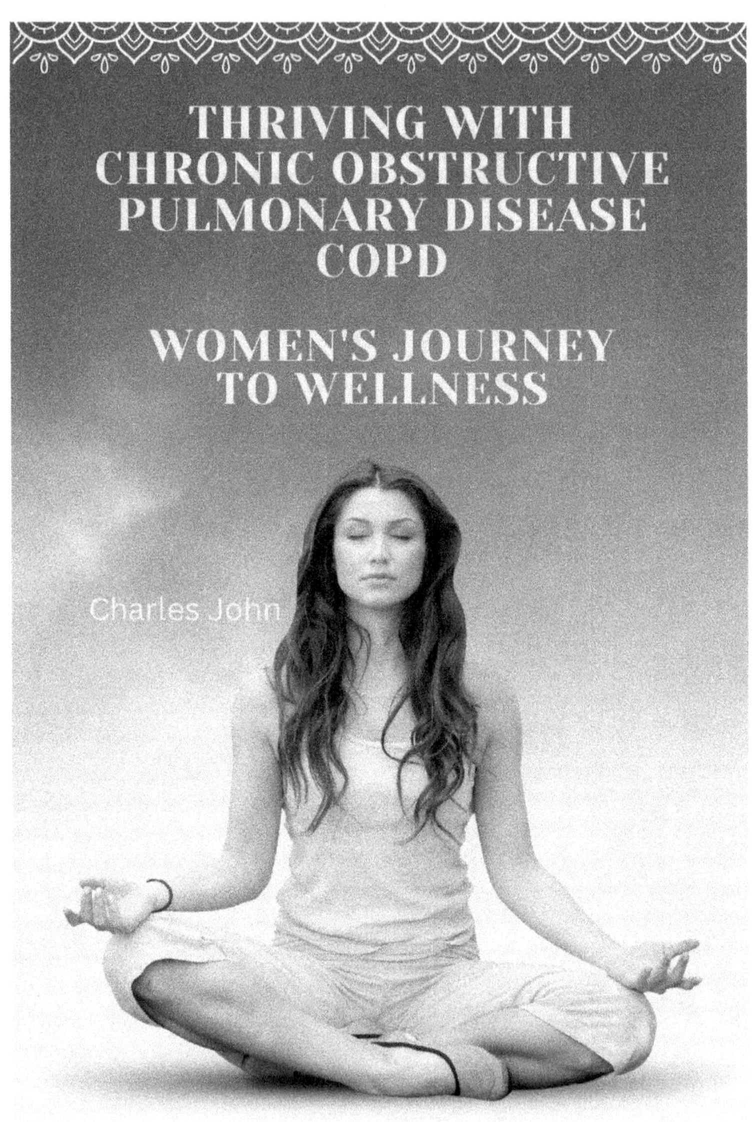

THRIVING WITH
CHRONIC OBSTRUCTIVE
PULMONARY DISEASE
COPD

WOMEN'S JOURNEY
TO WELLNESS

Charles John

TABLE OF CONTENTS

INTRODUCTION

CHAPTER 1

Signs And Symptoms Of COPD

Chapter 2

What Is Bronchitis Chronica?

Emphysema

CHAPTER 3

Women with Chronic Obstructive Pulmonary Disease (COPD)

Men, Women, and the Variations in COPD

The Effects of Marketing and Smoking on the Risk to Women

Other Ways That COPD Affects Women Besides Tobacco

How Do Women With COPD Get Treated?

Will A Lung Transplant Be Necessary If I Have Copd?

CHAPTER 4

Natural Home Cures For COPD

Ten COPD-related supplements

INTRODUCTION

The long-term inflammatory lung condition known as chronic obstructive pulmonary disease (COPD) results in restricted lung airflow. Breathing problems, coughing up mucus (sputum), and wheezing are among the symptoms. Long-term exposure to irritating chemicals or particulate matter—most frequently from cigarette smoke—is usually the cause of it. Heart disease, lung cancer, and a host of other ailments are more likely to strike those with COPD.

COPD is mostly caused by two main conditions: emphysema and chronic bronchitis. Individuals with COPD may have varying degrees of severity for these two illnesses, which typically coexist.

Inflammation of the lining of the bronchial tubes, which transport air to and from the lungs' air sacs (alveoli), is known as chronic bronchitis. Sputum (mucus) output and a daily cough are its defining features.

The disease known as emphysema occurs when the lungs' alveoli, which are located at the end of their tiniest airways (bronchioles), are destroyed due to harmful exposure to cigarette smoke and other irritating chemicals and particulates.

Despite being a progressive illness that worsens with time, COPD is curable. Most COPD patients can obtain good symptom control, a high quality of life, and a lower chance of developing other related disorders with appropriate care.

CHAPTER 1

Signs And Symptoms Of COPD

The symptoms of COPD frequently take time to manifest, especially if smoking persists, and they usually increase after major lung damage has occurred.

COPD symptoms and indicators could include:

•Breathing difficulty, especially when moving around
•Sighing
•Tightness in the chest
•A persistent cough that may discharge clear, white, yellow, or greenish mucus, or sputum

•Recurring infections of the respiratory system
•Absence of vigor
•Intentional loss of weight (latter phases)
•Swelling in the feet, legs, or ankles

Exacerbations are episodes in which a person with COPD's symptoms worsen beyond what they typically are on a daily basis and last for a few days or longer.

When To Visit A Physician

Speak with your doctor if your symptoms are not getting better or are becoming worse after therapy, or if you experience any infection-related symptoms like fever or a change in your sputum.

If you are experiencing significant blueness of the lips or nail beds (cyanosis), a fast heartbeat, difficulty breathing, or dizziness and difficulty focusing, get medical attention right once.

Reasons

Tobacco usage is the primary cause of COPD in developed nations. People who live in unadventurous dwellings and are frequently exposed to fuel fumes from cooking and heating commonly develop chronic obstructive pulmonary disease (COPD).

While many smokers with extended smoking histories may experience impaired lung function, only a small percentage of chronic smokers acquire clinically evident COPD. Some smokers experience less frequent lung problems. Until a more comprehensive evaluation is conducted, they can be incorrectly labeled as having COPD.

The Impact On Your Lungs

Air passes through two large tubes (bronchi) in your lungs and down your windpipe (trachea). These tubes in your lungs split into numerous smaller tubes (bronchioles), which finish in clusters of microscopic air sacs (alveoli), much like a tree's branches do.

Very thin walls, called capillaries, brim with small blood vessels that make up the air sacs. As you breathe in, oxygen from the surrounding air enters these blood vessels and travels throughout your body. The gas carbon dioxide, a waste product of metabolism, is exhaled simultaneously.

To expel air from your body, your lungs rely on the bronchial tubes' and air sacs' inherent elasticity. They become less elastic and over expand as a result of COPD, which traps some air in your lungs when you exhale.

Emphysema
Emphysema Click to enlarge
Chronisis Chronisis View larger image
reasons for blockage of the airways

A blockage of the airway can be caused by asthma. The delicate alveolar walls and elastic fibers are destroyed by this lung illness. When you exhale, your small airways constrict, making it harder for air to leave your lungs.

extended bronchitis. This illness causes inflammation and narrowing of the bronchial tubes, as well as increased mucus production in the lungs, which can obstruct the airways even more. In an attempt to clear your airways, you start to cough constantly.
Smoke from cigarettes and other irritants
Long-term cigarette smoking is the primary cause of lung damage in the great majority of COPD patients. However, as not all smokers get COPD, there are probably other factors at work as well, such as a hereditary vulnerability to the disease.

Cigarette, pipe, and secondhand smoke, air pollution, and exposure to dust, smoke, or fumes at work are some other irritants that can cause COPD.

Lack Of Alpha-1-antitrypsin

About 1% of COPD patients have low levels of a protein called alpha-1-antitrypsin (AAt), which is caused by a genetic condition. To aid in lung protection, AAt is produced in the liver and released into the bloodstream. A deficit in alpha-1-antitrypsin may result in lung disease, liver disease, or both.

Treatment options for adults with COPD associated with AAt deficiency are similar to those offered to patients with more common forms of COPD. Furthermore, in certain cases, treatment involves substituting the absent AAt protein, perhaps averting additional lung injury.

Factors at risk

COPD risk factors include:

exposure to smoke from tobacco. The main cause of COPD is a history of long-term cigarette smoking. Your risk increases with the number of years and packs you smoke. Those who smoke marijuana, cigars, pipes, or other tobacco products, as well as those who are frequently around secondhand smoke, may also be at risk.

those who suffer from asthma. A persistent inflammatory airway illness called asthma may increase the chance of getting COPD. The risk of COPD is further increased when smoking and asthma coexist.
Industrial exposure to chemicals and dust. Your lungs may become irritated and inflamed if you are exposed to chemical fumes, vapors, or dust on a regular basis at work.

exposure to fuel combustion byproducts. People in underdeveloped nations who live in dwellings with inadequate ventilation and are exposed to the fumes from burning fuel for cooking and heating are more likely to develop COPD.

genetics. Some COPD instances are caused by the rare genetic condition alpha-1-antitrypsin deficiency. There are probably more hereditary factors that increase a smoker's risk of developing the illness.

Difficulties

A number of issues can arise from COPD, such as:

infections of the respiratory system. It is more common for people with COPD to get pneumonia, the flu, and colds. Any respiratory infection has the potential to worsen lung tissue damage and make breathing considerably more difficult.

cardiac issues. Heart disease, including heart attacks, can be made more likely by COPD for unclear reasons.

carcinoma of the lung. The risk of lung cancer is increased in those with COPD. elevated intracranial pressure in the lungs. Pulmonary hypertension, or elevated blood pressure in the arteries supplying blood to the lungs, is a possible side effect of COPD.

Depression. Breathing problems may prevent you from engaging in enjoyable activities. Furthermore, managing a severe disease may have a role in the emergence of depression.

Avoidance
In contrast to many illnesses, COPD usually has a known origin, a well-defined course for prevention, and methods for delaying the disease's course. Since most cases are directly linked to cigarette smoking, quitting

smoking early on or never smoking is the greatest method to prevent COPD.

This straightforward advice might not appear so straightforward to long-term smokers, particularly if you've made numerous unsuccessful attempts to stop smoking. But don't give up on quitting. Locating a smoke cessation program that can assist you in quitting permanently is essential. This is your best opportunity to lessen lung damage.

Another risk factor for COPD is exposure to chemical dusts and fumes at work. Speak with your supervisor about the best ways to protect yourself, such as wearing respiratory protection equipment, if you work with these kinds of lung irritants.

***The following actions can assist in preventing COPD-related complications**:*

Give up smoking to lower your risk of lung cancer and heart disease.

To lower your risk of contracting some infections, consider getting vaccinated against pneumococcal pneumonia and the flu each year. If you feel hopeless or depressed, or if you suspect you may be suffering from depression, consult your physician.

Chapter 2

What Is Bronchitis Chronica?

Inflammation of the breathing tubes is called bronchitis. These are the bronchi, or airways. In addition to other alterations, this inflammation results in excessive mucus production. Different kinds of bronchitis exist. Acute and chronic, however, are the most prevalent.

Long-term bronchial irritation is known as chronic bronchitis. It is typical of smokers. Lung infections are common in people with chronic bronchitis. They also experience worsening symptoms with bouts of acute bronchitis.

To qualify as long-term bronchitis:

For two years in a row, you must have a cough and mucus on most days for at least three months of the year.
It is necessary to rule out other possible explanations of the symptoms, such as lung disorders or tuberculosis.
Individuals with chronic obstructive pulmonary disease (COPD) also have chronic bronchitis. This is a broad category of lung conditions, among which is chronic bronchitis. Breathing issues may result from these illnesses' ability to obstruct lung airflow. Emphysema and chronic bronchitis are the two diseases associated with COPD most commonly.

Why does chronic bronchitis occur?
There is no virus or bacteria that causes chronic bronchitis. The majority of experts concur that smoking cigarettes is the primary cause of chronic bronchitis. Your

workplace and air pollution can also be factors. If you smoke, this is especially true.

Symptoms of pneumonia may coexist with other lung conditions, including:

*Inhalation
*Emphysema pulmonary
*Lung scarring (pulmonary fibrosis)
*A sinus infection
*Tuberculosis
*Infections of the upper respiratory tract

What signs of chronic bronchitis are present?

The most typical signs of chronic bronchitis are listed below. However, symptoms can vary slightly from person to person.

Among the symptoms could be:

Cough, also referred to as smoker's cough

Mucus coughing (expectoration)
Sighing
Discomfort in the chest

Before experiencing dyspnea, people with chronic bronchitis frequently cough and produce mucus for years.

Long-term bronchitis may result in:

Infirmity
frequent and serious infections affecting your respiratory system
breathing tube narrowing and blockage (bronchi)
Breathing difficulties.

Additional signs and symptoms could be:

Bluish complexion, lips, and fingernails due to low oxygen levels
breathing while making crackling and wheezing noises
enlarged feet

heart attack

Chronic bronchitis might mimic other lung Diseases or health issues in its symptoms. Consult your physician for a diagnosis.

How is the diagnosis of chronic bronchitis made?

Together with a thorough medical history, your healthcare professional will do a physical examination. The following tests could be ordered by him or her:

Tests for pulmonary function

The capacity of your lungs to pump air into and out of them is measured by these examinations. Frequently, the examinations are conducted using specialized breathing apparatuses. They could consist of:

Spirometry. This examination measures your lung function using a spirometer. It is among the most straightforward and widely used lung function tests. Any or all of the following purposes could make use of it:

To measure the capacity of your lungs to take in, hold, and transfer air.
To monitor a pulmonary condition.
To assess the effectiveness of the treatment.
To determine the severity of your lung ailment.
To determine if the lung illness you have is obstructive or restrictive.

Restrictive implies that you will breathe in less air. If something is obstructive, less air will leave your lungs.
peak flow meter. This test determines how quickly you can expel air from your lungs. The major airways in the lungs become narrowed because of inflammation and mucus. The air exiting the lungs moves more slowly as a result. It is quantifiable using a peak flow monitor. This assessment is crucial for determining how effectively your illness is being managed.

Blood gas in the arterial system
Your blood's carbon dioxide and oxygen content will be measured using this test. It gauges your blood's acidity as well.

The pulse oximeter

A tiny device called an oximeter gauges how much oxygen is in your blood. A tiny sensor is affixed to a finger or toe using tape or a clip in order to obtain this measurement. The sensor has a little red light that illuminates when the machine is activated. The red light does not heat up, and the sensor is painless.

X-ray of the chest
Images of your internal organs, bones, and tissues—including your lungs—are captured by this exam.

CT scan
This imaging test creates images of the body by combining computer technology and X-rays. Any aspect of the body, including the bones, muscles, fat, and organs, can be seen in great detail on a CT scan. Compared to standard X-rays, CT scans provide more detail.

How can one treat persistent bronchitis?

The goal of treating chronic bronchitis is to address both the symptoms and the underlying cause. It might consist of:

Giving up smoking.
Keeping away from other lung irritants and secondhand smoking.
Taking medications orally to help remove mucus and open airways.
Using medications for inhalation, such as steroids and bronchodilators.

Obtaining oxygen from transportable reservoirs.
Undergoing lung reduction surgery to remove lung damage.
Receiving a lung transplant, infrequently.
Adding moisture to the atmosphere.

pulmonary rehabilitation to teach you how to manage your breathing issues and continue being active. The essentials of chronic bronchitis. Inflammation of the bronchi (breathing tubes) is called bronchitis. Although there are many varieties of bronchitis, acute and chronic forms are the most prevalent.

A common component of chronic obstructive pulmonary disease (COPD) is chronic bronchitis. These are a set of lung conditions that result in breathing difficulties and airflow obstruction. Cigarette smoking is the primary cause of chronic bronchitis. Your workplace and air pollution can also be factors.

This illness results in a cough that is frequently referred to as a smoker's cough. You also experience chest pain, wheeze, and mucus-filled coughing. These could deteriorate over time and cause serious breathing issues.

Chronic bronchitis is diagnosed with functional pulmonary function tests. Blood, breathing, and imaging tests may also be used to see how severe the problem is and watch it over time. Controlling symptoms is the aim of treatment in order to lead a more comfortable life. Giving up smoking is a crucial component of treatment.

Here are some pointers to make the most of your appointment with your doctor:

•Be clear about your goals and the purpose of your visit.

•Make a list of the questions you would like answered before your visit.

•Ask questions and make sure you remember the information your healthcare provider gives you by bringing a companion.

•Note any new medications, treatments, or tests, as well as the name of any new diagnosis, at the visit. Note down any additional instructions you receive from your healthcare practitioner as well.

•Understand the benefits of every new medication or treatment that is prescribed to you. Be aware of the adverse effects as well.

•Inquire about alternative treatments for your problem.

•Understanding the possible meaning of the test or procedure is recommended.

•Understand what to anticipate in the event that you skip the medication, test, or operation.

•If you have a follow-up appointment, write down the date, time, and purpose for that visit.

•Know how you can contact your healthcare practitioner if you have questions.

Emphysema

Emphysema is a lung ailment that causes shortness of breath. In persons with emphysema, the air sacs in the lungs (alveoli) are destroyed. Over time, the inner walls of the air sacs weaken and rupture — creating bigger air holes instead of many small ones. This reduces the surface area of the lungs and, in turn, the amount of oxygen that reaches your circulation.

Fresh, oxygen-rich air cannot enter because old air becomes caught in the malfunctioning alveoli during exhalation. The majority of emphysema patients also have chronic bronchitis. An ongoing cough is a symptom of chronic bronchitis, an inflammation of the bronchial tubes, which are the tubes that convey air to your lungs.

Emphysema and chronic bronchitis are two disorders that make up chronic obstructive pulmonary disease (COPD). The main cause of COPD is smoking. Treatment may reduce the progression of COPD, but it can't reverse the damage.

Signs and symptoms

Emphysema can go for years without presenting any symptoms or indicators. Breathlessness is the primary symptom of emphysema, and it typically starts slowly. Breathlessness is a symptom that you may begin to avoid, so it doesn't become an issue until it starts to interfere with everyday activities. Breathlessness eventually results from emphysema, even when you're at rest.

When To Visit A Physician

If you've been experiencing unexplained dyspnea for a few months, see your doctor, particularly if it's becoming worse or becoming more of a hindrance to your everyday activities. Don't brush it off by convincing yourself that it's just a sign of aging or being overweight. Seek emergency medical assistance if:

You can't even climb stairs because you're out of breath.
When you exert yourself, your fingernails or lips turn gray or blue.
You lack mental awareness.
Make an appointment.

Reasons

Emphysema is primarily brought on by prolonged exposure to airborne allergens, such as:

•Smoke from tobacco
S•moke from marijuana
•Air contamination
•Dust and chemical fumes

Emphysema is infrequently brought on by a hereditary lack of a protein that shields the lungs' elastic components. Alpha-1-antitrypsin deficiency emphysema is the term for it.

Factors at risk

The following variables raise your chance of having emphysema:

✓ Smoking.

Although those who smoke cigarettes are more likely to acquire emphysema, those who smoke cigars or pipes may also be at risk. The longer a smoker has smoked and the more tobacco they have smoked, the higher the risk is for all smoker types.

Years old. The majority of individuals with tobacco-related emphysema start to exhibit signs of the illness between the ages of 40 and 60, despite the fact that the lung damage associated with the condition develops gradually.

✓Exposure to smoke in the vicinity. Tobacco smoke that you unintentionally breathe in from someone else's cigarette, pipe, or cigar is referred to as secondhand smoke, also known as passive or ambient tobacco smoke. The chance of developing emphysema increases when exposed to secondhand smoke.

✓Air pollution or dust exposure during work. Emphysema is more likely to develop if you breathe in fumes from specific chemicals or dust from wood, grain, cotton,

or mining materials. If you smoke, your risk increases even more.
exposure to pollution both outside and indoors. Emphysema risk is increased by breathing both outside and interior contaminants, such as car exhaust, or fumes from heating fuel.

Difficulties

Additionally, those with emphysema have a higher chance of developing:

Pulmonary Collapse (pneumothorax)

People with severe emphysema already have severely impaired lung function, so a collapsed lung can be life-threatening. This is rare, but when it does happen, it's serious.

Cardiac Issues

Pressure in the arteries that carry blood from the heart to the lungs might rise as a result of emphysema. A condition known as cor pulmonale may result from this, wherein a portion of the heart weakens and enlarges.

Bullae

Bullae are large holes in the lungs. Bullae, which are empty areas in the lungs, can develop in certain emphysema patients. They may enlarge to the size of half the lung. Giant bullae not only limit the lung's ability to expand, but they also raise the possibility of pneumothorax.

Avoidance

Avoid inhaling secondhand smoke and quitting smoking to prevent emphysema. If you deal with dust or chemical vapors at work, wear a mask to protect your lungs.

CHAPTER 3

Women with Chronic Obstructive Pulmonary Disease (COPD)

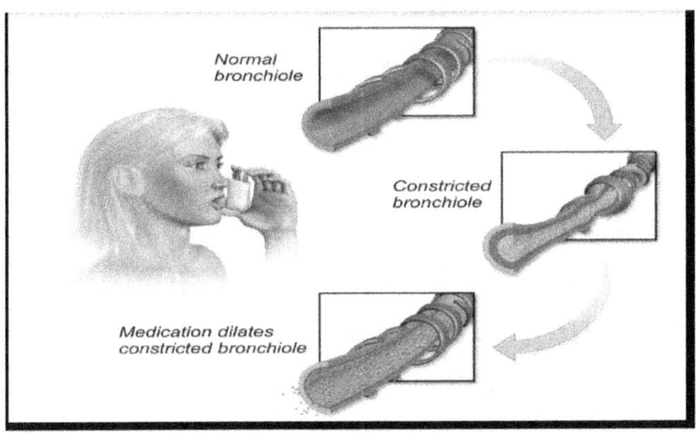

Unfortunately, Chronic Obstructive Pulmonary Disease (COPD), which affects over ten million Americans, is currently the third most common cause of mortality in the country. Compared to men, the number of women with COPD is rising more quickly. Women's COPD mortality and prevalence have increased significantly over the past few decades, matching those of men.

The effects of COPD on men and women vary. Women with COPD experience worse quality of life related to symptoms and increased dyspnea. Compared to males, women experience anxiety and depressive symptoms more frequently. According to a recent study, 1 in 4 COPD patients experienced persistent depression symptoms over a three-year period, and having a feminine gender identity was linked to significantly higher risks of persistent depressed symptoms. Although COPD and other smoking-related disorders frequently coexist, the associated diseases typically differ in individuals with COPD who are male or female.

It's possible that women are more vulnerable to the negative effects of tobacco smoke. Compared to men, women who smoke see a faster loss in lung function. The bulk of COPD patients who are not smokers are female, and they seem to be more susceptible to non-tobacco causes of the disease. The use of biomass fuels for cooking in underdeveloped nations may be the cause of a large number of non-smoking COPD cases, and women may be more susceptible to environmental toxins and secondhand smoke than men are.

Uncertainty surrounds the causes of these variations. Due to their smaller lungs than men's, women may be more exposed to the negative effects of cigarette smoke for the same amount of smoking. Additionally, there are variations in the kinds of cigarettes smoked. Menthol cigarettes are more popular among women, and they are very dangerous. It's also possible that males and women have different hormone environments. There is another genetic component.

Given these variations in COPD susceptibility and clinical presentation, it would seem that men and women would react differently to COPD conventional therapies. Regretfully, women have historically not participated extensively in COPD treatment trials, however this is starting to change. Women react to quitting smoking differently than men do, and their lung function improves more after stopping than it does for males, but they also struggle more to maintain their quitting habits.

In addition to the regrettable increased incidence of COPD in women, there is mounting evidence that women with COPD may need distinct treatment options due to their unique symptoms and risk factors. Drs. Megan Hardin, Barbara Cockrill, and Dawn DeMeo collaborate with you in the BWH Women's Lung Health Program to help you comprehend these distinctions and receive the finest care available.

Men, Women, and the Variations in COPD

Chronic obstructive pulmonary disease (COPD) is one of the illnesses that medical professionals are diagnosing and treating in women more frequently. COPD is one of several illnesses and ailments that manifest in women differently than in males. According to ongoing studies, COPD affects more women than males in the United States. The disease is also killing off more women than men. In actuality, the death rate from COPD is rising in women but down in males.

In general, women experience more severe COPD symptoms than men do. In addition, women are more likely than males to have flare-ups, or exacerbation of symptoms.

The Effects of Marketing and Smoking on the Risk to Women

When we examine how COPD affects women's health and quality of life, numerous factors come into play. But smoking is one of the main contributing factors. Nowadays, women smoke in the United States almost as much as males do. Nevertheless, studies reveal that compared to their male colleagues with COPD, women with the disease frequently smoke less.

Women's lungs may be more vulnerable to the harmful effects of cigarette smoking since their airways and lungs are frequently smaller than men's. Over the years, the tobacco business has increased the consumption of cigarettes among women, women of color, and women who identify as LGBTI.

"Slim" cigarettes were promoted to women in the 1960s and 1970s who wished to look trim and feminine. Communities of color were sold menthol cigarettes in the 1980s under the false impression that they were smoother and healthier—instead, they are more dangerous and addictive.

Tobacco companies targeted LGBTQ people in the 1990s in an effort to increase smoking rates within those communities. The companies linked their products to the AIDS research, women's rights movement, and music festivals primarily attended by communities of color through sponsorships, special promotions, and customer recruitment. It should come as no surprise that over 85% of Black smokers smoke menthol cigarettes, and that lesbian and bisexual girls smoke cigarettes at a rate nearly ten times higher than that of their heterosexual counterparts.

The greatest risk factor for developing COPD is tobacco use. Therefore, there will be an increase in the number of COPD diagnoses among women who smoke, especially among women in underrepresented communities.

Other Ways That COPD Affects Women Besides Tobacco

Other ways that COPD may affect women's health include co-occurring conditions, restrictions, or potentially harmful outcomes:

The Osteoporosis

This prevalent bone disease deteriorates the strength, structure, and tissue of bones. There may be more fractures as a result. About half of the persons with COPD also have osteoporosis, and osteoporosis is considerably more common in my female patients than in my male ones. One of the risk factors for osteoporosis is smoking. It can weaken bones by lowering their blood supply, which limits their capacity to produce new cells and stops the body from absorbing adequate bone making calcium.

Stress, Depression, and Anxiety

These disorders can impact how people think, feel, and handle daily activities. Research reveals that women with COPD may be more prone to feel anxiety and sadness when compared to both males with COPD and women without COPD. One reason may be because women with COPD sometimes have more shortness of breath than males with COPD. Unequal demands of household and childcare obligations may result in higher levels of stress in women with COPD compared to males.

Hospitalizations

Women account for a larger number of COPD-related hospital admissions and inpatient fatalities than do men with COPD.

Activity Limitations

Studies suggest women with COPD report a worse ability to exercise and worse overall health-related quality of life compared to men with the illness.

Underdiagnosed and Misdiagnosed is Common

Research alludes to the possibility that COPD may be underdiagnosed in women. Even though many women have both illnesses, I often get referrals from women who were informed they had asthma but not COPD. Owing to this prejudice, women may receive a diagnosis of the illness later on, when there may be fewer alternatives for therapy.

The most popular diagnostic for COPD, a spirometry test, may be less likely to be provided to women with symptoms than to men. This is an easy test: inhale deeply, then exhale as forcefully as you can into a machine that records the amount of air you release and the speed at which you do it. When a woman comes in with COPD symptoms or is at risk for the illness but doesn't currently have symptoms, I run this test on her first. I think there would be a reduction in the time it takes to diagnose COPD in women if more medical professionals performed spirometry tests on them.

The process of diagnosis may also involve additional testing. Among them are:

•A Computed Tomography (CT) Scan or Radiography Of The Chest.

These exams produce images of the heart and lungs that may reveal COPD symptoms.

•Test For Arterial Blood Gas.

This test evaluates blood carbon dioxide and oxygen levels. It can assist in determining whether a lady requires oxygen therapy or not.

•Oximetry Of The Pulse.

This test uses a painless clip on a finger or earlobe to monitor blood oxygen levels. It has the ability to detect oxygen deficiency in females.

How Do Women With COPD Get Treated?

If a patient smokes, always have a conversation with them about quitting, regardless of their gender. It is extremely crucial for smokers with COPD to give up. It may aid in delaying the illness's course. Furthermore, studies indicate that women with COPD gain even more than males do from giving up smoking. One year after quitting smoking, women's breathing improves twice as much as men's does.

Recommend free smoking cessation hotlines, like this one from the PA-DOH (1-800-QUIT-NOW), to patients with COPD who smoke.

Additionally, refer smokers with COPD to the Health Center's Smoking Cessation Program for behavioral counseling. Prescribe or suggest FDA-approved drugs to help smokers quit smoking to those who are not pregnant. Don't recommend e-cigarettes to someone who wants to stop smoking since they have no place in the quitting process. Numerous individuals have had lasting cessation of smoking thanks to the combination of behavioral counseling and medication.

Treatment for COPD is generally the same for men and women. I regularly recommend the following courses of treatment to COPD patients:

Medications that reduce inflammation and expand airways. These may include bronchodilators, additional anti-inflammatory medications, and inhaled corticosteroids.

rehabilitation of the lungs. With this care, patients can manage their COPD both physically and psychologically. Exercise, advice on managing the illness, and nutritional counseling are a few examples.

oxygen treatment. This can help patients receive more oxygen than they would from their regular breathing and can greatly facilitate daily tasks like walking and housework.

yearly flu shots in addition, if the patient hasn't had the injection earlier, a pneumonia vaccine. For those with COPD, pneumonia and the flu can both result in life-threatening respiratory difficulties.

Will A Lung Transplant Be Necessary If I Have Copd?

α-1 antitrypsin deficiency emphysema and COPD continue to be two of the main reasons for lung transplantation. Patients may be eligible for lung transplantation if all other treatment options—such as oxygen therapy, noninvasive ventilation, rehabilitation, and lung volume reduction—have been tried and tested or are not feasible.

CHAPTER 4

Natural Home Cures For COPD

Treatment for COPD can make it better. Coughing, excessive mucus production, and other symptoms can be relieved at home. The lung ailment known as chronic obstructive pulmonary disease (COPD) is persistent. Airflow into and out of the lungs is restricted by COPD. Because of their propensity for dyspnea, people with the illness may find it difficult to exercise and carry out daily tasks.

While there isn't a treatment for COPD at the moment, there are a number of natural remedies that can help clear the airways and enhance a person's quality of life. This book explains how people can manage their COPD at home with the use of vitamins, essential oils, and changes in lifestyle.

At-home treatments for COPD

The following natural therapies and at-home cures for COPD can help patients control their symptoms and delay the course of the illness:

1. Give up smoking
Giving up smoking can delay the progression of COPD.
About 90% of COPD-related deaths in the US are caused by smoking, which is also the most common cause of the disease.
Smoke from tobacco products affects the lungs' airways. The airways narrow as a result of inflammation and blockage, making it harder for air to enter and exit.

A recent review found that smoking increases lung function decline, comorbidities, and death risk in individuals with COPD. The efficacy of inhaled steroid medicines, which physicians utilize to treat severe COPD, may also be diminished by smoking. The best thing a smoker with COPD can do to reduce the disease's progression is to give up smoking. For step-by-step instructions on quitting, people can visit smokefree.gov or consult a doctor.

2. Upgrade the home's air quality
People with COPD may find it harder to breathe in some household irritants. Typical irritants consist of:

Varnishes and paints
Chemical-based cleaning supplies
Dust, tobacco smoke, chemicals, and pet dander
Homeowners can enhance the quality of the air by:

minimizing exposure to common household contaminants
utilizing an air filtering system and opening windows to enhance ventilation, as well as

routinely cleaning air filters to stop the spread of mold and mildew
vacuuming and clearing clutter to stop dust from accumulating and washing bed linens once a week to lower dust mite populations

3. Engage in breathing techniques
Breathing exercises are intended to alleviate the symptoms of COPD by strengthening the muscles involved in breathing and enhancing an individual's capacity for exercise. In a 2012 Cochrane comprehensive review, groups of COPD patients who performed breathing exercises for four to fifteen weeks were compared to those who did not.

Among the breathing techniques were:

breathing with pursed lips. This is the process of breathing in via the nose and out through firmly closed lips.
breathing with the diaphragm. This entails drawing in the diaphragm to facilitate

deeper breathing. When breathing in, the belly obviously swells, and when breathing out, it noticeably contracts.

Pranayama. This method of controlled breathing is frequently used in yoga exercises. During pranayama, one focuses on the parts of the body used for breathing.

Researchers did not find any differences in quality of life or symptoms like dyspnea; nevertheless, those who practiced breathing exercises reported better exercise tolerance. Those with COPD who find it difficult to exercise may find relief through breathing exercises.

4. Control your stress levels

Stress on an emotional level might impair immunity and raise the possibility of COPD flare-ups.

Sudden exacerbations of symptoms are a possible side effect of COPD. The likelihood of flare-ups may be heightened by anxiety and sadness. Using stress-reduction techniques will enhance overall health.

One investigationAccording to a Trusted Source study, individuals with COPD who also struggled with anxiety or depression had a higher chance of returning to the hospital within 30 days after discharge. Stress on an emotional level can impair immunity, raising the possibility of respiratory infections.

Reducing emotional suffering may be aided by mindfulness meditation. An 8-week mindfulness meditation course improved respiratory rate in COPD patients as compared to the control group, according to a small-scale 2015 study (Trusted Source). After six lessons, participants also reported having better emotional functioning.

5. Continue to weigh a healthy amount
Individuals with COPD who are underweight are more likely to die from the

disease than those who are overweight. Researchers are constantly looking into how obesity affects the prognosis for COPD.

Underweight COPD patients are more likely to encounter:

Weakening in the muscles used for breathing.
Diminished capacity for exercise
Diminished ability to breathe

A balanced diet can aid persons with COPD by enhancing lung function, per a recent review. Additionally, a balanced diet is good for the heart and metabolism. Underweight individuals may benefit most from a diet rich in calories, protein, and unsaturated fats.

When paired with exercise, this kind of diet helps build muscle and gives one more energy. Nevertheless, more extensive research is required before scientists can fully comprehend the advantages of this diet for COPD patients.

6. Build up your muscle mass
Breathing becomes more difficult during exercise for many persons with COPD. However, symptoms like exhaustion and muscle weakness can get worse if you don't exercise.

People with COPD may benefit from the following exercises to strengthen their muscles and boost their capacity for exercise:

training intervals. This means doing high- and low-intensity workouts back-to-back. People with severe COPD can benefit from interval training because it strengthens muscles without taxing the heart or lungs. Strengthening exercises. This increases muscle size and strength by applying resistance using weights, resistance bands, and an individual's body weight. Increasing the strength of your lower body muscles can assist alleviate dyspnea.

When someone starts to lose fitness, exercise gets harder and their lung function could get worse. Therefore, for maximum benefits, people should begin an exercise regimen early.

7. Exercises in the water

Exercise may be more challenging for people with COPD due to bone or muscular disorders. People with COPD may find water activities easier and more bearable because they put less strain on the body.

According to a 2013 study, exercising in the water may improve one's quality of life and ability to exercise. Exercise on the water proved to be more beneficial for COPD patients with physical impairments than either land-based exercise or no exercise at all. The peculiar qualities of water, which provide resistance to raise exercise intensity and maintain body weight through buoyancy, may be the cause of these effects, the researchers hypothesized.

By lowering symptoms and regulating inflammation, a variety of vitamins can assist manage COPD symptoms. Among the supplements for COPD are:

8. Calcium
A lack of vitamin D may worsen the body's capacity to eliminate microorganisms and cause inflammation of the airways, according to a reliable source.

A review from 2015 Low levels of vitamin D were shown to be common in patients with severe COPD, according to Trusted Source. Supplemental vitamin D may help with flare-ups and some COPD symptoms.

Vitamin D supplements are available online and at pharmacies.

9. Creatine with Co-enzyme Q10
Natural substances called creatine and coenzyme Q10 (CoQ10) help provide the body's cells with energy.

A 2013 investigationA study conducted by Trusted Source examined the potential benefits of coQ10 and creatine supplements on COPD symptoms in individuals suffering from chronic respiratory failure.

Those who took both CoQ10 and creatine supplements for two months reported better quality of life, less breathlessness, better activity tolerance, and fewer flare-ups. CoQ10 can be purchased online or at pharmacies.

Essential oils
Additionally, people can utilize essential oils to unclog their airways and remove lung mucus. Essential oils can be applied topically or diffused using a carrier oil to

dilute them. Among the essential oils for COPD are:

10. Oil of eucalyptus
The oil of eucalyptus has anti-inflammatory qualities.
Eucalyptol is a naturally occurring chemical found in eucalyptus oil. People with COPD may benefit from eucalyptol in the following ways:

possesses anti-inflammatory and antioxidant qualities
decreases mucus production and aids in the removal of mucus from the lungs by opening up the airways in the lungs.
keeps moderate to severe COPD flare-ups at bay. According to the findings of one study, Trusted Source recommends mixing 12 drops of eucalyptus oil with 150 milliliters of boiling water and taking a three-times-daily sniff. Online, there is a large selection of eucalyptus oils.

11. Standardized Myrtol
An essential oil called standardized is made from eucalyptus, pine, and lime.

According to a comprehensive analysis of 15 randomized controlled trials (RCTs), standardized is a secure and successful treatment for COPD and chronic bronchitis. But more extensive, superior RCTs are required.

When to visit a physician

If someone exhibits any of the following signs of a COPD exacerbation, they should consult a physician:

•Increased dyspnea
increased production of mucus compared to usual yellow, green, or brown mucus that is stickier or thicker than typical fever
symptoms of the flu and cold
heightened fatigue

A severe exacerbation of COPD is indicated by specific signs and symptoms. If someone has any of the following, they should contact emergency services straight away:

breathing difficulties, chest pain, bluish lips or fingers
agitation or confusion fatigue
Early intervention can lessen the chance of acquiring more difficulties from COPD exacerbations.

In summary, managing COPD can be challenging due to its chronic nature. Certain home treatments, including exercise, breathing exercises, nutritional supplements, and essential oils, can help people manage their symptoms at home.

A person has to consult their doctor if their COPD symptoms worsen.

Ten COPD-related supplements

Emphysema, refractory asthma, and chronic bronchitis are among the chronic lung disorders together referred to as chronic obstructive pulmonary disease, or COPD. Numerous dietary supplements and treatments may lessen the symptoms of COPD.

Breathing becomes more and more difficult for those with COPD. They might have tightness in the chest, wheezing, and coughing, among other symptoms. For the 15.7 million people in the US who have been diagnosed with COPD, nutrition is crucial.

The COPD Foundation states that because breathing requires more work than normal, patients with COPD may require 430–720 extra calories per day. Indeed, malnutrition affects 25–40%Trusted Source of individuals with COPD, which negatively impacts their prognosis in the long run.

Currently, COPD cannot be cured. But according to the American Lung Association, those who have respiratory issues may benefit from following a high-fat, low-carb diet. In addition, there are a number of supplements and home treatments that patients with COPD can attempt to complement their medical care and assist in managing their illness. To find out more, continue reading.

Vitamins

InvestigatorsThe vitamins listed below are recommended for treating and supporting COPD, according to Trusted Source:

1. Calcium
Low vitamin D levels are common in COPD patients. Supplementing with vitamin D may improve lung function.

For COPD patients, taking vitamin D3 supplements can also help prevent mild to severe flare-ups.

2. Calcium
Reduced vitamin C levels are associated with increased mucus production, wheezing, and dyspnea.

3. E. vitamin
Individuals with COPD who are going through a flare-up typically have lower vitamin E levels than those whose COPD is stable.

Long-term usage of vitamin E supplements may help prevent COPD, according to other research.

4. Vitamin A
According to an earlier evaluation, a study indicated that those with the highest vitamin A intake had a 52% decreased risk of developing COPD.

Minerals

The following minerals have been shown by researchers to be beneficial for treating and supporting COPD:

5. Magnesium
While magnesium helps the lungs function, several COPD drugs might make it difficult for the body to absorb magnesium.

Additionally, people with COPD should use caution when using magnesium supplements. It may have negative effects and conflict with some medications.

6. Calcium
Although some COPD drugs may cause the body to lose calcium, calcium can help the lungs function. This emphasizes how crucial it is for those who have COPD to think about including more foods high in calcium in their diet.

It can be required for someone to take a calcium supplement if their diet isn't enough to meet their calcium demands.

Additional supplements

The following extra supplements have been found by researchers to be beneficial for treating and supporting COPD:

7. Fatty acids omega-3
Increasing omega-3 fatty acid consumption may help COPD patients feel less inflammatory. Omega-3s can be found in fish, seeds, and nuts, but some individuals

prefer to take fish oil supplements to ensure their intake of this nutrient is adequate.

8. dietary fiber
A decreased risk of COPD may result from eating more dietary fiberTrusted Source.

9. Teas made with herbs
The following teas are popular among COPD sufferers as a way to lessen symptoms:

Lemon balm tea, lime tea, linseed tea, sage tea, thyme tea, marshmallow tea, rosehip tea, and mint tea
As a matter of fact, studies have indicated that consuming green tea at least twice daily may lower the chance of getting COPD.

10. Curcumin
Curcumin, which is found in turmeric, is occasionally referred to as a natural anti-inflammatory.

According to some research, it might aid in the treatment of COPD-related airway inflammation.

When to visit a physician

Because COPD is progressive and chronic, it does not go away and usually gets worse over time. To monitor and control their health, people with COPD must schedule frequent checkups with their physician. Prescription medications can help persons with COPD manage their symptoms, even if they cannot stop the progressive loss of respiratory ability.

Additionally, individuals with COPD can avoid diseases that could result in serious problems by receiving regular flu shots. These factors make routine medical treatment necessary for COPD patients.
While taking supplements can be beneficial for COPD patients, it is important for them to discuss all of their supplement intake

with a physician or other trained healthcare provider.

Medication for COPD may interact and become ineffective with some vitamins, minerals, herbs, and other products. They might have adverse consequences as well.

In brief, chronic lung disease (COPD) is a severe medical illness.

While there isn't a cure for this illness yet, patients can manage their symptoms with the use of medical intervention. Taking nutritional and herbal supplements for COPD may also aid in the treatment of symptoms. One should consider the usage of supplements with a physician or other healthcare provider prior to taking any.

Periodically, individuals with chronic obstructive pulmonary disease (COPD) may experience flare-ups, or an increase in symptoms. Bronchodilators, corticosteroids, antibiotics, oxygen therapy, and ventilation are among the treatments available for exacerbations.

The umbrella term for a collection of chronic lung conditions is COPD. The illness usually worsens with time, and some of the symptoms are as follows:

breathing difficulties that wheeze
coughing up too much mucus
tiredness and tightness in the chest
Occasionally, people with COPD may discover that their current symptoms abruptly worsen or that they develop new ones. These times are known by medical professionals as flare-ups or exacerbations.

A change in weather, an infection, or exposure to irritants or allergens can all cause an aggravation in some people.

Discover a few of the possibilities for managing a COPD exacerbation in this book. We also go over the significance of managing exacerbations, the circumstances in which hospitalization would be required, and some advice on how to avoid exacerbations.

Options for exacerbation treatment
In general, it is best for someone to start therapy for a COPD exacerbation as soon as possible. There are numerous possibilities for treatment, such as:

Bronchodilators

A COPD exacerbation's symptoms can be lessened by opening the airways using a bronchodilator.

Medication called a bronchodilator helps to open up the airways by relaxing the muscles surrounding them. Albuterol is one of the bronchodilators that physicians administer to patients with COPD the most frequently.

Increased wheezing, shortness of breath, or chest tightness may be signs of a COPD exacerbation. These symptoms may be lessened by using bronchodilators or other medications that dilate the airways.

Bronchodilators are usually supplied as a liquid or as an inhaler device. In order to take the liquid form, one needs to utilize a device known as a nebulizer to transform the liquid into an aerosol or mist that can be inhaled.

Use of a bronchodilator may cause shakiness, headaches, and an accelerated heart rate.

Corticosteroids

An increase in airway and lung inflammation may be the cause of a COPD exacerbation. Corticosteroids can aid in symptom relief and inflammation reduction. There are various types of corticosteroids.